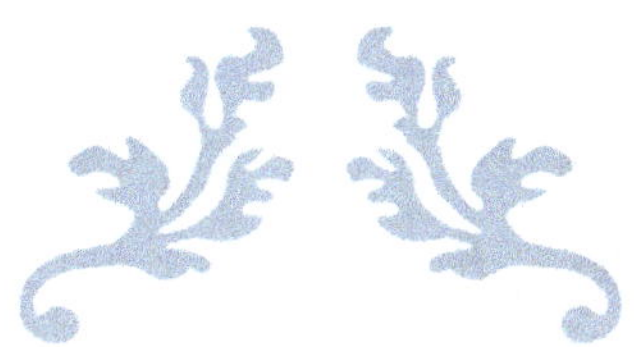

GALVESTON DIET FOR MENOPAUSAL WOMEN

Delicious Anti-Inflammatory Recipes and Effortless Weight Loss with Intermittent Fasting Guide to a Healthier, Happier You

LORA W. BRAXTON

CONTENTS:

Chapter 1: Introduction

Why do women gain weight in menopause?

Why Do Women Gain Weight in Menopause?

Introducing the Galveston Diet

Chapter 2: Anti-Inflammation and Intermittent Fasting

The Connection Between Chronic Inflammation, Menopause, and Weight Gain.

Understanding the power of anti-inflammatory foods.

Understanding the Science of IF

Chapter 3: Choosing Your Path with the Galveston Diet

Exploring the Different Levels of the Program: Foundations, Momentum, and Transformation.

Customizing your Galveston Diet

Setting realistic goals and expectations for success

Chapter 4: Anti-Inflammatory Food Playground - Nourishing Your Body with Delicious Choices

Building your plate with nutrient-rich, inflammation-fighting foods.

Shopping smart for the Galveston Diet - essential grocery staples and pantry must-haves.

Delicious and Satisfying Recipe Ideas for Breakfast, Lunch, Dinner, and Snacks.

Breakfast

Lunch

Dinner

Snacks

Chapter 5: Mastering Intermittent

Exploring different intermittent fasting schedules: 16:8, 5:2, and beyond.

Tips for navigating social events, travel, and unexpected situations.

Overcoming hunger cravings and staying motivated during fasting periods.

Chapter 7: Conquering Challenges and Roadblocks

Addressing weight plateaus, hormonal fluctuations, and social setbacks.

Maintaining commitment and motivation in the long run

Chapter 7: Sustainable Strategies for Maintaining Momentum

Practical Tips for Everyday Life.

Adapting the Journey to the Stages of Life

Laying the Groundwork for Healthy Aging

CONCLUSION

DEDICATION

This book is dedicated to you, warrior lady whose spirit knows no age. Every day, you face the light, determined to soar beyond limits, especially the whispers of weight gain that might precede menopause. You seek independence in your body, unrestricted mobility, and a fire kept alive by vitality.

This is a tribute to your fortitude, tenacity, and unwillingness to be defined by numbers on a scale. You realize that fitness is a symphony of well-being - a clear mind, a strong heart, a body that moves with the elegance of a dancer and the force of a mountain.

Hi, we hope you enjoyed this book! We'd really appreciate your honest feedback to help us improve. Would you mind leaving a review

PART 1: UNDERSTANDING THE GALVESTON DIET

Chapter 1: Introduction

Why do women gain weight in menopause?

Menopause is a key turning point in a woman's life, not just emotionally and hormonally, but also physiologically. Weight gain is one of the most prevalent side effects of this change, which can leave many people unhappy and confused.

Understanding the "why" of menopausal weight gain is essential for women to handle this transition with confidence and understanding. It's not as simple as "eating more and moving less," as popular narratives indicate. Instead, it's a complicated combination of hormonal changes, metabolic alterations, and lifestyle variables that all contribute to weight increase at this age.

The Hormonal Symphony

Hormones are chemical messengers that regulate many body activities. There are about 50 distinct hormones in your body, and many of them gradually drop with age. The two principal female hormones are estrogen and progesterone, and low amounts cause perimenopause and, eventually, menopause.

Low estrogen has a variety of effects on your body, one of which is a slower metabolism. Your metabolism is the mechanism by which you transform the calories you eat into energy. A sluggish metabolism means you don't burn calories as quickly, making weight loss more difficult.

Maintaining the same exercise and eating habits throughout menopause increases your chances of gaining weight because your metabolism isn't as effective. That weight is more prone to accumulate around your midsection.

Hormonal fluctuations also have an impact on your body composition. Without modifying your behaviors, you may begin to lose muscle mass and acquire fat, causing your metabolism to decrease and making it easier to gain weight.

These hormonal changes are a primary cause of menopausal weight increase, but there are other variables at work as well. Your level of physical activity, food, and even the amount of sleep you get each night can all have an impact on your body weight. Estrogen, the female hormonal orchestra's conductor, is important in controlling metabolism, fat distribution, and hunger. Estrogen maintains fat largely retained in the hips and thighs throughout a woman's reproductive years, generating a pear-shaped body type. It also aids in the maintenance of insulin sensitivity, maintaining proper blood sugar homeostasis.

However, as menopause approaches, estrogen levels drop. This hormone change disrupts the orchestra, resulting in numerous consequences:

Fat Redistribution: A lack of estrogen causes the body to store fat in a different way, causing a shift from the lower body to the belly, resulting in an apple-shaped body type. This visceral fat is more hazardous since it increases the risk of heart disease, diabetes, and other chronic diseases.

Metabolic Slowdown: Estrogen also affects how quickly your body burns calories, a process known as metabolic rate. The engine of metabolism sputters as it ages, leading you to burn less calories at rest and during exercise. This means that you can gain weight even if you continue to eat and exercise normally.

Greater Appetite: Changes in other hormones that govern appetite and satiety, such as leptin and ghrelin, can contribute to greater cravings and a less efficient sensation of fullness after meals. This can lead to overeating and more weight gain.

Beyond Hormones

While hormones play an important role, other lifestyle variables might increase or alleviate menopausal weight gain. These include:

Stress: Prolonged stress causes the stress hormone cortisol to be released, which encourages the accumulation of fat around the abdomen. It might be good to find healthy ways to handle stress, such as via yoga, meditation, or spending time in nature.

Sleep Disruption: Inadequate sleep can cause hormonal abnormalities that alter hunger and metabolism. Prioritizing sleep hygiene and sticking to a regular sleep pattern can help.

Reduced Physical Activity: As energy and motivation levels diminish after menopause, so does physical activity. Regular exercise, even if it is as simple as walking or swimming, is essential for preserving muscle mass, increasing metabolism, and controlling weight.

bad dietary choices heavy in sugar, processed foods, and bad fats can all lead to weight gain. A balanced diet rich in fruits, vegetables, whole grains, and lean protein is essential.

Why Do Women Gain Weight in Menopause?

How many calories have I ingested and burned?

These are two questions that many individuals will ask themselves when attempting to reach a specific "goal weight." Unfortunately, the questions boil down the complexities of weight reduction and health management to a simple addition and subtraction of calorie intake vs activity. However, counting calories is not the only way to lose weight and, more importantly, keep it off.

While knowing the "why" of menopausal weight gain is critical, figuring out "how" to control it brings its own set of difficulties. Many women turn to traditional weight loss methods, only to discover that they are frustratingly useless and even detrimental at this time of life. This is why:

1. The Calorie Counting Conundrum: In menopause, the usual "calories in, calories out" approach frequently falls short. Focusing simply on calorie restriction might overlook hormonal and metabolic changes. Excessive calorie restriction might reduce metabolic rate, making it even more difficult to lose or maintain weight loss.

2. The Exercise Mysteries: While exercise is still important for overall health and weight control, menopausal women confront special problems. Intense exercise routines may be stressful, raising cortisol levels and sabotaging weight reduction goals. High-impact activities may aggravate joint discomfort, a typical complaint after menopause, discouraging long-term participation.

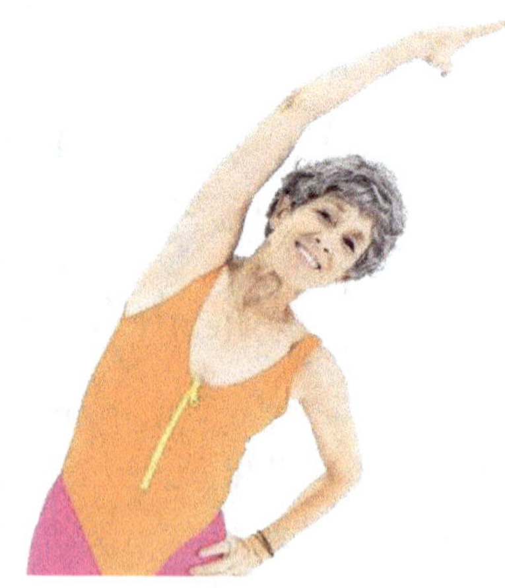

3. The Trendy Diet Crash diets and restrictive eating programs may produce rapid results, but they are unlikely to be sustainable in the long run. Depriving your body of necessary nutrients can cause more hormonal disruption, unhealthy appetites, and rebound weight gain.

4. The One-Size-Fits-All Trap: Many traditional weight reduction procedures are developed for a general population, neglecting menopausal women's special needs. They overlook the unique hormonal changes, metabolic slowness, and changed body composition that lead to weight gain at this time.

5. The Ageism Barrier: Messages from society and the media that promote unattainable beauty standards and ideal body types can be especially demotivating for women in menopause. These messages frequently fail to recognize the normal changes that occur with age, which can lead to emotions of guilt and frustration that stymie weight loss efforts.

Changing the Narrative

Rather than pursuing unachievable standards, the emphasis in menopause should shift to appropriate weight control that promotes overall well-being. This includes the following:

Taking a customized approach: Understanding the distinct hormonal and metabolic shifts that every woman goes through and modifying plans accordingly.

Prioritize anti-inflammatory foods: Prioritizing nutrient-rich, complete meals that fight inflammation and promote hormonal balance.

Mindful eating and intuitive movement: Practicing mindful eating and mild exercise routines that increase body awareness and satisfaction.

Stress management and sleep hygiene: Using ways to manage stress, prioritize sleep, and enhance emotional well-being.

Connecting with other menopausal women and receiving expert advice from healthcare professionals and registered dietitians who specialize in hormonal health can help you build a supportive group.

Introducing the Galveston Diet

Navigating the difficulties of standard weight reduction techniques in menopause might feel like you're lost in a maze. But what if a light shine through, giving a comprehensive road to better health, hormonal balance, and general well-being in addition to weight management? This is where the Galveston Diet comes into play, a ray of hope devised exclusively for women at this critical juncture in their lives

Anti-Inflammation, Intermittent Fasting, and Individualized Support are the Empowerment Pillars.

The Galveston Diet, unlike one-size-fits-all solutions, is built on three strong pillars:

1. Anti-Inflammation: Body and Mind Nourishment: The notion of controlling inflammation is central to the diet. Chronic inflammation, which is sometimes aggravated by hormonal changes after menopause, contributes significantly to weight gain, insulin resistance, and other health issues. Whole, unprocessed foods high in antioxidants and anti-inflammatory characteristics, including as fruits and vegetables, lean protein, healthy fats, and whole grains, are emphasized in the Galveston Diet.

This emphasis on providing the body with the proper fuel aids in the reduction of inflammation, the improvement of metabolic health, and the promotion of general well-being.

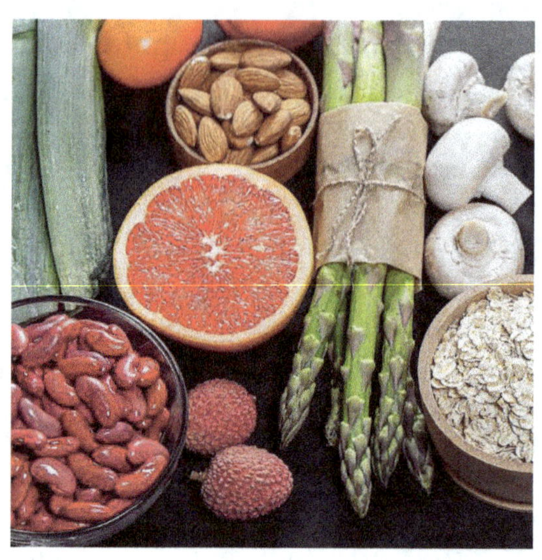

2. Intermittent Fasting: Re-establishing Rhythms and Revitalizing Metabolism: Another important pillar is intermittent fasting, which entails alternate periods of eating and fasting. This personalized technique helps to reset the body's normal metabolic cycles, increase fat burning, and enhance insulin sensitivity. Intermittent fasting has been proven in studies to be especially beneficial for menopausal women, helping to prevent the age-related metabolic slowdown and decrease belly fat.

3. Individualized Assistance: Finding Your Way, Achieving Your Goals: The Galveston Diet understands that each woman's journey is unique. It provides several degrees of assistance and supervision, allowing individuals to select the path that best meets their requirements and interests. The program allows women to adapt their path to their objectives and speed, whether it's the Foundations level for gentle assistance, the Momentum level for a more organized approach, or the Transformation level for full support.

The Galveston Diet is about more than just losing weight. It is a comprehensive strategy that focuses on:

- **Hormonal Balance**: By treating inflammation and promoting good metabolic function, the diet can help to balance hormones and relieve menopausal symptoms, resulting in more energy, better sleep, and fewer mood swings.

- **Mindful Eating:** The program promotes mindful eating practices, assisting women in developing a healthy connection with food and developing lasting habits for long-term weight management.

- **Stress Management:** The Galveston Diet encourages methods for reducing stress and fostering emotional well-being in order to maximize the path towards a better lifestyle, acknowledging the link between stress and weight gain.

Building Confidence: The Galveston Diet allows women to prioritize their health and enjoy their changing bodies with its tailored approach and focus on total well-being, generating a sense of confidence and self-acceptance.

Chapter 2: Anti-Inflammation and Intermittent Fasting

The Connection Between Chronic Inflammation, Menopause, and Weight Gain.

Menopause signals a turning point not just in hormones, but also in your body's quiet war, which is fueled by the flames of chronic inflammation. While weight gain may appear to be as easy as "eating more and moving less," it is typically this hidden fire that plays the villain, upsetting your metabolism and laying the scene for extra pounds.

In this chapter, we'll look closely at the relationship between chronic inflammation, menopause, and weight gain. We'll reveal the processes at work, decipher the function of hormone fluctuations, and provide you with the information you need to confront this silent adversary and restore your metabolic health.

The Inflammation Flames

Chronic inflammation isn't just the odd flare-up after an injury; it's a low-grade fire that's fed by a variety of causes. The terrain transforms considerably after menopause, providing situations that feed the fires of inflammation even more:

Estrogen Retreat: A decrease in estrogen levels upsets your body's delicate balance of inflammatory indicators. Estrogen is generally a dampener, but its fall permits pro-inflammatory chemicals such as C-reactive protein (CRP) to proliferate.

Adipose Tissue Transformation: Fat distribution shifts when estrogen levels fall. Fat begins to migrate from the hips and thighs (pear-shaped) to the belly (apple-shaped). This visceral fat isn't only different in appearance; it's also more physiologically active, producing inflammatory signals that fuel the fire.

Stress and Sleep Disruption: The emotional ups and downs of menopause are frequently accompanied by chronic stress and interrupted sleep habits. These elements fuel the inflammatory fire, resulting in a vicious cycle that contributes to weight gain.

The Domino Effect of Weight Gain

Inflammation doesn't simply sit there and stew; it actively disrupts your body's metabolic process, tilting the balances in favor of weight gain:

- Inflammation impairs your body's capacity to use insulin properly, resulting in blood sugar increases and increased fat deposition, particularly in the belly.

- Metabolic Stagnation: The inflammatory storm slows your metabolic rate, which means your body consumes calories at a slower rate, making it more difficult to maintain or lose weight.

- Inflammation can disturb the delicate dance of appetite-regulating hormones such as leptin and ghrelin, leading to increased desires for sugary and processed foods and prolonging the cycle of inflammation and weight gain.

Tools for Fighting the Rebellion

Understanding your adversary is half the fight. Let us now empower ourselves with techniques to quell the fires of inflammation and restore our metabolic health:

Embrace an anti-inflammatory diet rich in colorful fruits and vegetables, omega-3 fatty acids, healthy grains, and lean protein. These foods are high in antioxidants and phytonutrients, which naturally reduce inflammation.

Fasting as a Metabolic Reset: Intermittent fasting, such as the 16:8 approach, can help reduce CRP levels and increase insulin sensitivity, lowering inflammation and assisting with weight control.

Warriors of Stress Management: Yoga, meditation, and other stress-relieving activities assist decrease cortisol, a stress hormone that has been linked to inflammation. Sleeping first strengthens your body's natural anti-inflammatory activities.

The Inflammation Quencher: Exercise Regular physical exercise, even short walks, can lower inflammatory indicators dramatically. Find things that you like and exercise your body with purpose.

Understanding the power of anti-inflammatory foods.

Inflammation is the body's reaction to potentially damaging stimuli like germs, damaged cells, or irritants. It entails a complicated biological process aimed at removing the source of cell harm, clearing away necrotic cells and tissues damaged by the initial insult, and inflammatory cells in the afflicted area.

Chronic inflammation occurs when the immune system's reaction lasts for a lengthy period of time, frequently without resolving. This persistent inflammation can cause tissue damage and contribute to the onset of chronic illnesses. Chronic inflammation can be exacerbated by lifestyle factors such as poor food, lack of exercise, stress, and environmental pollutants.

Anti-inflammatory foods contain chemicals that have the ability to decrease inflammation in the body. These foods are high in antioxidants, polyphenols, and other bioactive chemicals that reduce inflammation.

These hidden plant heroes aren't just tasty; they're also loaded with powerful chemicals that function wonders on a cellular level:

Antioxidants: These superfoods scavenge free radicals, the damaging chemicals that cause inflammation. Consider them small shields that safeguard your cells from the inflammatory maelstrom.

Phytonutrients: These distinct plant components have powerful anti-inflammatory capabilities. Certain berries contain anthocyanins, while spices like turmeric include curcumin, both of which are powerful anti-inflammatory agents.

Omega-3 Fatty Acids: Found in fatty fish, walnuts, and chia seeds, these beneficial fats not only lower inflammation but also boost heart health and cognitive function.

Some of the most important anti-inflammatory foods are:

- **Fruits and veggies:** Fruits and vegetables, which are high in vitamins, minerals, and antioxidants, have an important role in lowering inflammation. Berries, leafy greens, and cruciferous vegetables stand out in particular.

- **Fatty Fish:** Omega-3 fatty acids, which are found in fish such as salmon, mackerel, and sardines, have powerful anti-inflammatory properties.

- **Nuts and seeds:** Omega-3s and antioxidants are abundant in almonds, walnuts, flaxseeds, and chia seeds.

- Whole grains, such as brown rice, quinoa, and oats, include fiber and other nutrients that may aid in inflammation reduction.

- **Whole Grains:** Foods like brown rice, quinoa, and oats provide fiber and other nutrients that may help lower inflammation.

- **Herbs & Spices:** Due to their anti-inflammatory qualities, turmeric, ginger, garlic, and cinnamon are frequently utilized in traditional medicine.

Understanding the Science of IF

While anti-inflammatory meals provide your body with culinary cavalry, intermittent fasting (IF) is another potent weapon in your inventory. This technique, which is sometimes cloaked in mystery, may be a beneficial tool for women in menopause, aiding in hormone balance, increasing fat burning, and paving the path for a healthier you.

But, let's face it, intermittent fasting may be daunting. Missing meals? Are you having trouble with your metabolism? The worries are valid, but the advantages are worth considering. So, let us shine a light on this technique and reveal its potential to strengthen your menopausal journey.

IF, unlike typical calorie-counting regimens, emphasizes cycling between eating and fasting times. This is not about deprivation; it is about allowing your body to relax and restore its metabolic processes. Consider it a vacation for your digestive system, enabling it to focus on other critical duties such as cellular repair and hormone regulation.

The science underlying the magic is as follows:

Insulin Reset: When you eat, your body releases insulin to transport glucose (energy) into your cells. Insulin levels fall during fasting times, enabling your body to use stored fat for fuel. This can significantly increase fat burning, especially the stubborn belly fat that builds after menopause.

Hormonal Balance: Research suggests that IF can improve the delicate balance of hormones such as estrogen and insulin, potentially alleviating menopausal symptoms and encouraging healthy metabolic function.

Cellular Rejuvenation: Fasting triggers processes such as autophagy, in which your body cleanses itself by eliminating damaged cells, potentially increasing cellular health and lifespan.

Discovering Your Fasting Flow

The beauty of IF is its adaptability. There is no one-size-fits-all approach, so you may select a style that best suits your lifestyle and interests. Here are some popular choices:

- **16:8 Method:** This involves fasting for 16 hours (usually overnight and into the morning) and eating within an 8-hour window. This is a gentle approach for beginners.

- **5:2 Method:** Eat normally for five days, then limit your calorie consumption to 500-600 on two non-consecutive days.

- **Eat-Stop-Eat:** Once or twice a week, fast for 24 hours. This is more difficult, but it may yield faster results.

The Benefits of IF

Improved Insulin Sensitivity: Because it lowers insulin levels and promotes fat burning, IF can minimize your chance of developing type 2 diabetes, which is a significant worry during menopause.

Enhanced Energy Levels: Fasting's metabolic transition to fat burning can deliver continuous energy throughout the day, leaving you feeling less lethargic and more energized.

Improves Cognitive Function: Research suggests that IF might increase brain function, memory, and attention, thereby minimizing cognitive decline linked with menopause.

Stress Reduction: IF can increase your body's relaxation response, possibly lowering stress and enhancing mood, both of which are useful allies when managing menopausal changes.

Chapter 3: Choosing Your Path with the Galveston Diet

Exploring the Different Levels of the Program: Foundations, Momentum, and Transformation.

Foundations

Consider the Foundations level to be the robust base camp from where your trip will begin. It's great for people looking for a moderate introduction to the Galveston Diet's anti-inflammatory concepts and practices. Here's what to expect:

Gradual Transition: This level promotes a gradual transition to anti-inflammatory foods and attentive eating practices. You will be given detailed instructions on how to fill your plate with colorful veggies, fruits, healthy grains, and lean protein while progressively lowering pro-inflammatory items.

Fundamental Knowledge: The curriculum will teach you the basics of chronic inflammation, its relationship to menopause and weight gain, as well as the science behind anti-inflammatory foods and intermittent fasting.

Personalized Support: You'll get access to online tools, useful hints, and support communities to aid you along the way.

Momentum

The Momentum level is ideal for people looking for a more organized approach with additional assistance and accountability.

Tailored Meal Plans: You'll get personalized meal plans based on your preferences and calorie needs, with anti-inflammatory concepts and mindful eating practices incorporated.

Intermittent Fasting Guidance: Get professional advice on implementing several IF programs and determining which one best matches your lifestyle and maximizes outcomes.

Personalized Coaching: Receive the assistance of a professional coach who gives regular check-ins, inspiration, and personalized changes to your plan as needed.

Interactive Community: In a helpful forum, connect with other women on the same path and exchange experiences, advice, and words of support.

Transformation

The makeover level welcomes you with open arms if you're ready for a comprehensive lifestyle makeover. This all-encompassing curriculum goes deeper into all facets of holistic health and well-being:

Intensive Coaching: Receive individualized coaching sessions that cover diet, exercise, stress management, sleep hygiene, and emotional well-being, paving the way for long-term transformation.

Advanced Meal Planning: Receive personalized meal plans suited to your individual health goals and nutritional needs, as well as continuing assistance from a specialized nutritionist.

Mind-Body practices: Learn about yoga, meditation, and other mindfulness practices to help you manage stress, sleep better, and nurture inner peace.

Personalized Exercise Strategies: Work with a competent trainer to create a personalized exercise regimen that ensures safety and efficacy while optimizing outcomes.

Customizing your Galveston Diet

Customizing your experience for a smooth transition to health and well-being throughout menopause. While anti-inflammatory dietary concepts are at the heart of the program, you are free to paint your plate with bright brushstrokes of personal tastes. Consider the following alternatives:

Vegetarian and Vegan Delights: Adopt an anti-inflammatory vegetarian or vegan diet, incorporating plant-based protein sources such as lentils, beans, tofu, and tempeh with a rainbow of vegetables and fruits.

Gluten-Free Harmony: If gluten sensitivity is an issue for you, look into alternative grains like quinoa, buckwheat, and brown rice to keep your cuisine anti-inflammatory and tasty.

Paleo Precision: If the Paleo strategy appeals to you, focus on lean protein, fruits, vegetables, and nuts while limiting processed foods and grains and remaining anti-inflammatory.

Dairy Dance: Select from a variety of alternatives! Enjoy full-fat yogurt and cheese for their probiotic advantages, or experiment with lactose-free options while maintaining enough calcium intake through leafy greens and fortified meals.

Setting realistic goals and expectations for success

Setting realistic objectives and expectations is essential for navigating the road map to a successful menopause. Reject false expectations of overnight transformations in favor of attainable milestones that nourish your body, mind, and spirit.

Setting SMART Goals

Specific, Measurable, Achievable, Relevant, and Time-bound (SMART) goals serve as a guidepost to meaningful progress:

- Begin with reasonable objectives, such as introducing two anti-inflammatory fruits into your daily diet or walking for 30 minutes three times each week. As you develop confidence and velocity, gradually raise the difficulty.
- Instead of concentrating on eliminating specific foods, create objectives for developing healthy habits such as cooking at home twice a week or practicing mindful eating for 15 minutes everyday.

- **Celebrate Non-Scale Victories:** Keep track of your success away from the scale! Recognize more sleep, less stress, and more energy as wins that add to your overall well-being.

- **Reframe Obstacles as Opportunities:** Consider setbacks to be brief diversions rather than obstacles. Learn from their mistakes, modify your strategy, and keep going forward with newfound zeal.

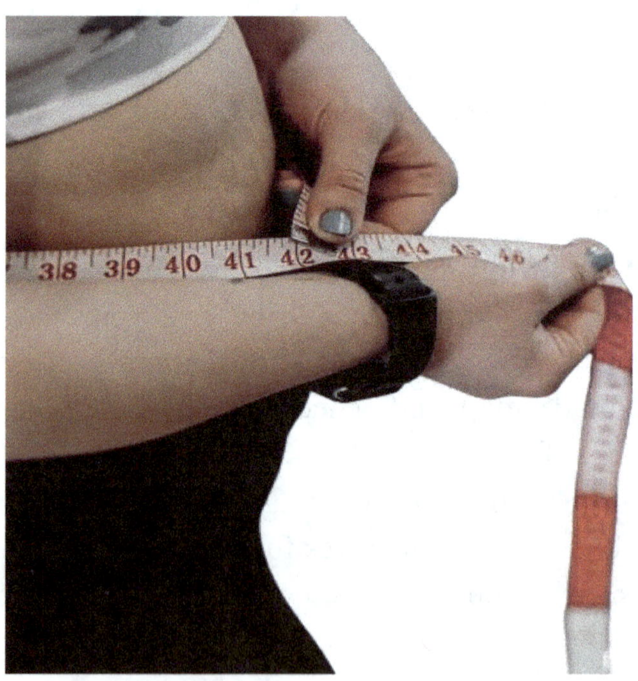

Here are some reasonable assumptions to have:

Anticipate Gradual Change and Long-Term Impact: Don't anticipate immediate miracles. The Galveston Diet focuses on developing long-term habits for health and well-being.

Weight Loss Plateaus: Weight loss may not be linear. Be patient with the process and celebrate plateaus as indicators that your body is adapting and responding.

Focus on Progress, Not Perfection: You will make mistakes. Don't let them dictate your path. Forgive yourself, learn from your mistakes, and recommit to your ambitions.

Every Milestone Should Be Celebrated: Recognize and appreciate every stride you take, no matter how tiny. Your success demonstrates your dedication and deserves to be recognized.

Seek Support and Community: Surround yourself with encouraging and guiding friends, family, and online groups who understand your path.

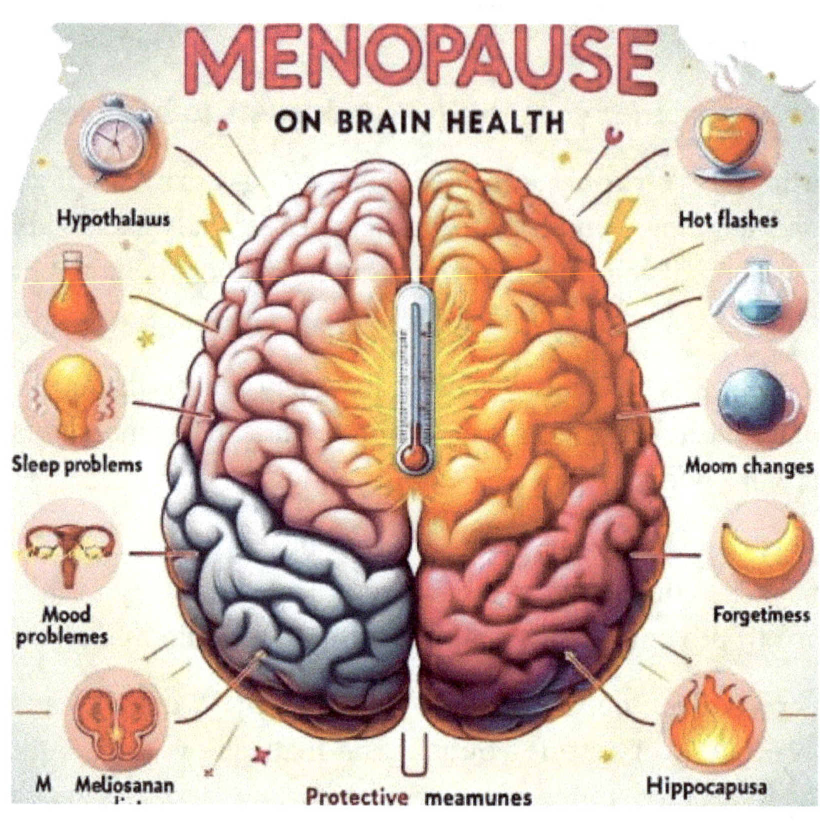

MENOPAUSE
ON BRAIN HEALTH
Hypothalaus
Hot flashes
Sleep problems
Moom changes
Mood problemes
Forgetiness
M Meliosanan
Hippocapusa
Protective meamunes

Chapter 4: Anti-Inflammatory Food Playground - Nourishing Your Body with Delicious Choices

Building your plate with nutrient-rich, inflammation-fighting foods.

The anti-inflammatory diet is a way of eating that is considered to help lower the risk of chronic inflammation-related disorders. An anti-inflammatory diet often contains lots of fruits and vegetables, lean protein, nuts, seeds, and healthy fats while avoiding packaged meals, sugary and salty foods, and processed red meat.

An anti-inflammatory diet is based on the premise that the foods you consume can help with inflammation in the body and lessen your risk of illnesses connected with chronic inflammation. An anti-inflammatory diet cannot be followed in a single method. You may mix it up and adjust the diet to your family's preferences and needs. However, there are certain anti-inflammatory diet principles you may follow:

- Every day, consume 5 to 9 servings of antioxidant-rich fruits and vegetables.
- Substitute lean poultry, fish, beans, and lentils for red meat.
- Replace butter and margarine with healthy fats like olive oil.
- Reduce your consumption of refined grains such as white bread, saltines, and pastries and replace them with more fiber-rich whole grains such as oats, quinoa, brown rice, and pasta.
- Instead of salt, season your meals with anti-inflammatory herbs such as garlic, ginger, and turmeric.
- Instead of deep frying, try baking, boiling, or braising your meal.

The anti-inflammatory diet is quite similar to the Mediterranean diet, which is another popular and health-promoting diet. Both diets emphasize nutrient-dense meals, healthy fats, and a variety of nutritious fruits and vegetables while reducing processed foods, red meat, and added sweets. The anti-inflammatory strategy focuses on incorporating fruits and vegetables that have been found to lower inflammation, such as dark leafy greens and blue and red fruits and vegetables including cherries, pomegranates, berries, and beets.

According to research, persons who consume a lot of vegetables, fruits, nuts, seeds, healthy oils, and seafood have a lower chance of developing inflammation-related disorders. Certain chemicals, such as antioxidants and omega-3 fatty acids, have anti-inflammatory properties.

Focus on Anti-Inflammatory Foods:

- Raspberries, blueberries, and blackberries
- Cherries
- Beets with Pomegranate
- Broccoli
- Cauliflower

- Bruxelles sprouts
- Greens with dark leaves (spinach, kale, chard)
- Nuts and seeds, particularly walnuts
- Nut butters made from natural ingredients
- Avocado
- Olive oil with olives
- Fish, particularly salmon and tuna
- Lentils, chickpeas, and other beans are examples of legumes.
- Quinoa, whole-wheat bread, and brown rice are examples of whole grains.
- Eggs
- sweet potatoes
- Fruits of citrus
- Herbs, garlic, and spices
- Greek yogurt and kefir

Shopping smart for the Galveston Diet - essential grocery staples and pantry must-haves.

Conquering the Galveston Diet begins in the grocery store aisles, not the kitchen. Navigating the shelves amid a sea of labels and options might be intimidating, but don't worry! This chapter will teach you how to be a savvy shopper, stocking your pantry with anti-inflammatory powerhouses and laying the groundwork for tasty, health-promoting meals.

Fresh Favorites for Your Fridge

Consider your refrigerator to be a lush landscape brimming with natural delights. Stock it with the following items for daily anti-inflammatory doses:

Leafy Green Brigade: Leafy greens such as kale, spinach, and arugula are high in antioxidants and phytonutrients. Pre-wash them and have them ready to put into salads, sandwiches, or smoothies.

Crunchy Cruciferous Crew: Broccoli, cauliflower, and Brussels sprouts have a gratifying crunch and are a potent source of anti-inflammatory nutrients. They may be roasted with olive oil and seasonings, steamed for a light side dish, or blended into creamy soups.

Bell Pepper Powerhouse: Bell peppers, which range in color from bright red to sunny yellow, are high in antioxidants and vitamin C. They may be sliced for nibbling, chopped into stir-fries, or roasted for a smokey sweetness.

Berrylicious Bunch: Berries including blueberries, strawberries, and raspberries are antioxidant powerhouses that are overflowing with flavor and ideal for on-the-go snacking, topping yogurts, or blending into refreshing smoothies.

Citrusy Sunkissed Squad: Oranges, grapefruits, and lemons offer a zesty flavor to your meals while also providing vitamin C and anti-inflammatory potency. Squeeze them into water, add them to marinades, or eat them as a refreshing after-meal snack.

Essentials for Everyday Use

A well-stocked pantry is your hidden weapon, offering easy access to nutritious ingredients for quick and delicious meals. Allow these culinary superstars to be your culinary allies:

Whole Grains for Longevity: Brown rice, quinoa, and oats provide complex carbs, fiber, and important minerals. Cook them in batches so they're ready for bowls, stir-fries, or nutritious pancakes.

Nutty goodness: Walnuts, almonds, and chia seeds are anti-inflammatory powerhouses filled with omega-3 fatty acids and important minerals. Toss them into homemade granola or sprinkle them over salads or yogurt.

Spice Spectrum: Turmeric, ginger, garlic, and rosemary are powerful anti-inflammatory fighters. Experiment with different combinations to enhance flavor and increase the nutritional value of your meals.

Canned Beans and Lentils: These protein-packed powerhouses are cupboard mainstays for quick and inexpensive meals. Toss them with olive oil and seasonings for a hearty vegan protein boost in salads, soups, and stews.

Healthy Fats: Olive oil, avocado oil, and flaxseeds include healthy fats that are necessary for satiety, vitamin absorption, and heart health. Drizzle them on salads, cook with them, or incorporate them into smoothies for extra creaminess.

Label Literacy

Knowing how to read food labels protects you against sneaky sugars and pro-inflammatory chemicals. Take note of the following: Serving Size: Keep portion management in mind and adapt recipes appropriately.

Sugar Content: Choose goods with natural sugars derived from fruits and vegetables, and avoid added sugars disguised as other ingredients.

Sodium Levels: To counteract water retention and inflammation, use items with reduced sodium concentration.

Ingredient List: Prioritize items that have entire, recognized components and minimize those that contain a large list of additions and preservatives.

Beyond the Store

Consider these options for your health and the environment while replenishing your pantry:

Shop Seasonally and Locally: Buying locally helps your community and assures freshness. Choose seasonal fruits and vegetables for the best flavor and nutritious content.

Choose Organic: Consider going organic wherever feasible, especially for food that is prone to pesticide residues.

Reduce Food Waste: To reduce food waste, plan your meals, buy exactly what you need, and use leftovers creatively.

Delicious and Satisfying Recipe Ideas for Breakfast, Lunch, Dinner, and Snacks.

Breakfast

Hemp Seed and Avocado Toast Recipe

Prep time: 10 mins   Cooking: 0 mins   servings:4

Ingredients

- 4 slices whole wheat bread
- 2 avocados, ripe
- 2 tablespoons hemp seeds
- 1 lemon (juiced)
- Season with salt and pepper to taste.

Instructions

1. Toast the bread pieces in the oven or in a toaster.
2. Remove the pit from the avocados and scoop out the meat into a basin.

3. Mash the avocado with a fork and season with salt and pepper.
4. On each slice of bread, spread the avocado mixture.
5. On top of the avocado mixture, sprinkle hemp seeds.
6. Serve and have fun!

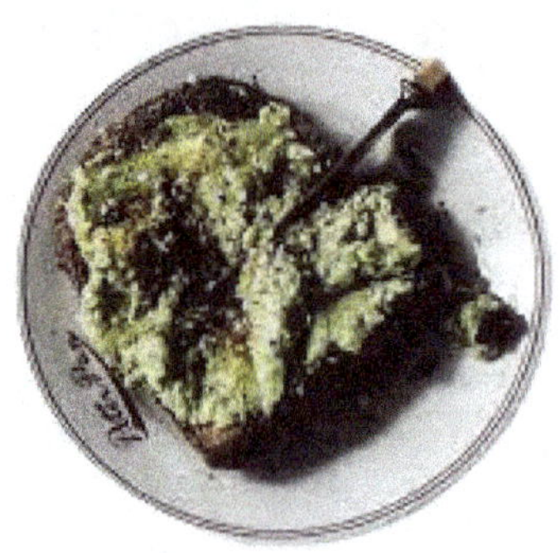

Berry and Spinach Smoothie Bowl

Prep time: 10 mins   Cooking: 0 mins   servings: 2

Ingredients

- 1 cup mixed frozen berries
- 1 banana, ripe
- 1 cup fresh spinach
- 1 cup almond milk

- 2 tbsp of chia seeds

Instructions

1. Blend till smooth the berries, banana, spinach, and almond milk.
2. Pour into serving dishes and sprinkle with chia seeds.

Nutritional Value (per serving)

- Calories: 250
- Fiber: 12g
- Protein: 5g

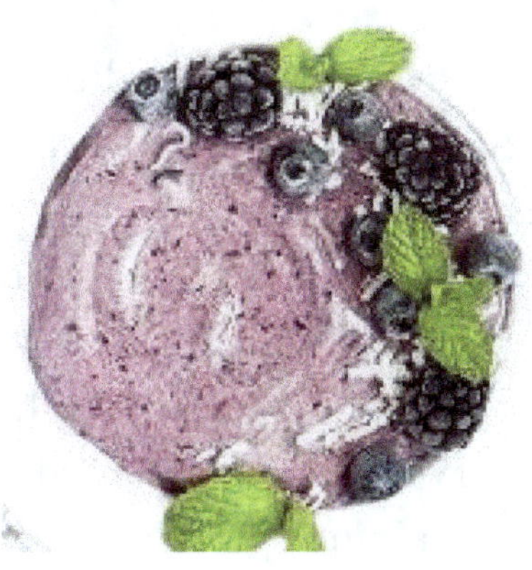

Turmeric and Ginger Oatmeal

Prep time: 5 mins   Cooking: 10 mins   servings:2

Ingredients

- 1 cup oats, old-fashioned
- 2 cups liquid (water or almond milk)
- 1 teaspoon turmeric powder
- 1/2 teaspoon ginger powder
- 1 teaspoon honey

Instructions

1. Bring the water to a boil in a medium saucepan.
2. Allow the ginger and turmeric root to soak for 2-3 minutes before adding the oats.
3. When the water turns a golden hue, toss in the oats and decrease the heat to medium-low.
4. Cook for 5-7 minutes, or until the liquid is mostly absorbed. Remove from heat after adding the raisins. Combine the remaining spices in a mixing bowl.
5. Transfer to a bowl and sprinkle with a teaspoon of coconut oil, pink salt, and a handful of coconut flakes.

Nutritional Value (per serving)

- Calories: 220
- Fiber: 5g
- Protein: 7g

Avocado and Salmon Toast

Prep time: 8 mins   Cooking: 2 mins   servings:2

Ingredients

- 2 slices whole wheat bread
- 1 mashed ripe avocado
- 4 oz. smoked salmon
- 1 teaspoon of lemon juice
- Garnish with fresh dill

Instructions

1. Toast some bread pieces.

2. On each piece, spread mashed avocado, then top with smoked salmon and sprinkle with lemon juice. Garnish with dill, if desired.

Nutritional Value (per serving)

- Calories: 300
- Fiber: 8g
- Protein: 15g

Quinoa Breakfast Bowl

Prep time: 15 mins   **Cooking: 15 mins**   **servings:2**

Ingredients

- 1 cup cooked quinoa
- 1/2 cup coconut milk
- 1 cup mixed berries
- 2 tablespoons shredded coconut
- 1 tablespoon maple syrup

Instructions

1. Heat cooked quinoa and coconut milk till heated.

2. Drizzle with maple syrup and top with mixed berries and shredded coconut.

Nutritional Value (per serving)

- Calories: 280
- Fiber: 6g
- Protein: 5g

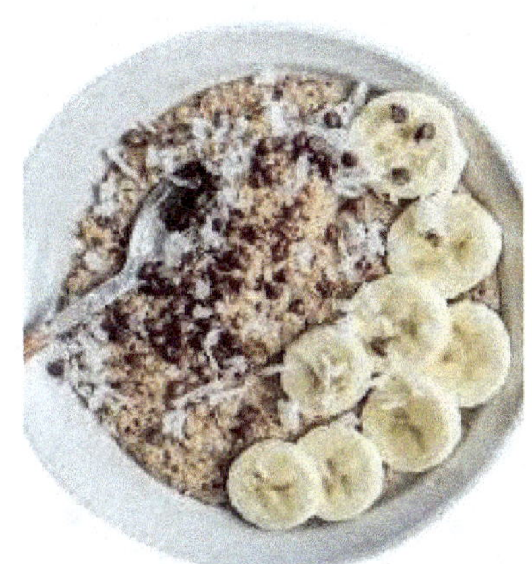

Chia Seed Pudding

Prep time: 5 mins   **Cooking: 0 mins**   **servings:2**

Ingredients

- 1/4 cup chia seeds

- 1 cup almond milk
- 1 teaspoon vanilla extract
- Fresh fruit for topping
- 1 tablespoon chopped nuts

Instructions

1. Mix chia seeds, almond milk, and vanilla extract. Refrigerate for at least 4 hours or overnight.
2. Top with fresh fruit and chopped nuts before serving.

Nutritional Value (per serving)

- Calories: 180
- Fiber: 10g
- Protein: 5g

Sweet Potato and Kale Breakfast Hash

Prep time: 10 mins   **Cooking: 20 mins**   **servings:2**

Ingredients

- 1 tablespoon olive oil
- 1/2 medium onion

- 1 sweet potato, medium
- 2 cups of kale
- 6 eggs
- 1/2 cup cheddar or parmesan cheese, salt & pepper

Instructions

1. Preheat the oven to 425 degrees Fahrenheit. Cut the sweet potato into bite-sized pieces. Toss with olive oil and bake for 20-25 minutes, or until the potatoes are tender.
2. While the sweet potato is cooking, wash and toss the kale with olive oil. Add the kale to the baking sheet after the sweet potato has finished cooking for 10 minutes and allow them to finish cooking together.

3. Add olive oil to a pan while they finish cooking. Add the onion, cut into small pieces, to the pan. Cook until they are clear. When the onions are done, stir in the cooked sweet potatoes and kale.
4. In a separate dish, whisk together the eggs and pour over the veggies in the pan. While the egg begins to cook, stir constantly. Add the cheese and stir it in just before the eggs are done. If desired, top with more cheese.

5. That's all! My favorite toppings are arugula and fresh chopped tomatoes!

Nutritional Value (per serving)

- Calories: 320
- Fiber: 8g
- Protein: 10g

Green Tea and Matcha Smoothie

Prep time: 5 mins   Cooking: 0 mins   servings:2

Ingredients

- 1 cup brewed green tea, cooled
- 1 banana
- 1 tablespoon matcha powder
- 1/2 cup Greek yogurt
- Ice cubes

Instructions

1. Blend green tea, banana, matcha powder, Greek yogurt, and ice cubes until smooth.

Nutritional Value (per serving)

- Calories: 180
- Fiber: 4g
- Protein: 7g

Mango and Coconut Chia Parfait

Prep time: 10 mins   Cooking: 0 mins   servings:2

Ingredients

- 1/4 cup chia seeds
- 1 cup coconut milk
- 1 ripe mango, diced
- Granola for layering
- 1 tablespoon honey

Instructions

2. Chia seeds and coconut milk should be combined. Refrigerate until completely set.

3. Layer chia pudding, chopped mango, and granola in serving glasses. Drizzle with honey to finish.

Nutritional Value (per serving)

- Calories: 250
- Fiber: 8g
- Protein: 6g

Cauliflower and Kale Breakfast Wrap

Prep time: 15 mins   Cooking: 10 mins   servings:2

Ingredients

- 4 large eggs, beaten
- 1 cup cauliflower rice
- 1 cup kale, thinly sliced
- 2 whole-grain wraps
- 1 tablespoon olive oil

Instructions

1. Sauté cauliflower rice and kale in olive oil until tender.

2. Scramble eggs and fold into the cauliflower and kale mixture. Spoon into wraps.

Nutritional Value (per serving)

- Calories: 320
- Fiber: 6g
- Protein: 14g

Blueberry and Almond Overnight Oats

Prep time: 5 mins   Cooking: 0 mins   servings:2

Ingredients

- 1 cup rolled oats
- 1 cup almond milk
- 1/2 cup fresh blueberries
- 2 tablespoons almond butter
- 1 teaspoon maple syrup

Instructions

1. Mix rolled oats and almond milk, refrigerate overnight.

2. Top with blueberries, almond butter, and a drizzle of
   maple syrup before serving.

Nutritional Value (per serving)

- Calories: 280
- Fiber: 8g
- Protein: 9g

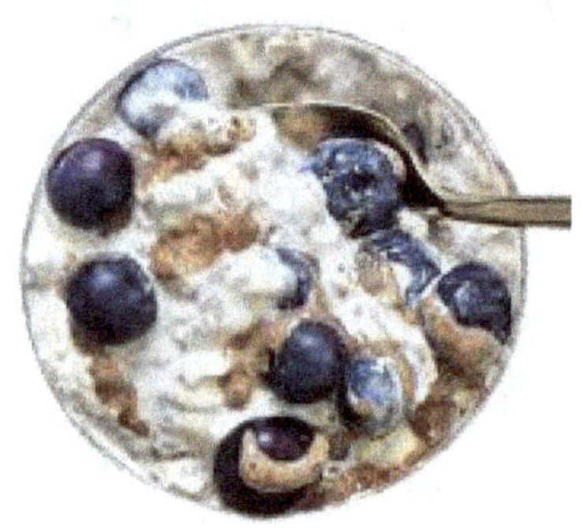

Lunch

Salmon and Avocado Salad

Prep time: 15 mins   Cooking: 10 mins   servings:2

INGREDIENTS

- 1.5 tbsp olive oil marinade/dressing
- 1 tbsp freshly squeezed lemon juice
- 0.5 tbsp (optional) red wine vinegar
- 0.5 tbsp chopped fresh parsley
- 1 teaspoon minced garlic
- 0.5 teaspoon oregano, dry
- To taste, 0.5 teaspoon salt and cracked pepper
- 500 g skinless salmon fillets (0.5 pound)

Salad

- 2 cups cleaned and dried Romaine (or Cos) lettuce leaves
- 0.5 large diced cucumber
- 1 Roma tomato, diced 1 red onion, sliced 1 avocado, sliced
- 0.25 cup crumbled feta cheese

- 0.17 cup sliced pitted Kalamata olives (or black olives)
- Serve with lemon wedges

INSTRUCTIONS

1. In a large mixing bowl, combine all of the marinade/dressing ingredients. Half of the marinade should be poured into a big, shallow dish. Refrigerate any leftover marinade to use as a dressing later.
2. Marinate the fish in the marinade. In a skillet or grill pan, heat 1 tablespoon oil over medium-high heat. Sear the salmon on both sides until it is crispy and cooked to your preference.
3. While the salmon is cooking, prepare the salad ingredients and combine them in a big salad dish.
4. Arrange salmon slices over salad. Drizzle with the last of the UNTOUCHED dressing. With lemon slices, serve.

Nutritional Value (per serving)

- Calories: 350
- Fiber: 8g
- Protein: 25g

Quinoa and Vegetable Stuffed Peppers

Prep time: 20 mins   Cooking: 25 mins   servings:4

Ingredients

- 1 cup quinoa, cooked
- 4 bell peppers, halved
- 1 cup black beans, cooked
- 1 cup corn kernels
- 1 cup cherry tomatoes, diced
- 1 teaspoon cumin powder
- 1/2 cup cilantro, chopped

Instructions

1. Preheat the oven to 375°F (190°C).
2. In a bowl, mix quinoa, black beans, corn, cherry tomatoes, cumin powder, and cilantro.
3. Stuff the bell peppers with the quinoa mixture and bake until peppers are tender.

Nutritional Value (per serving)

- Calories: 300
- Fiber: 10g

- Protein: 12g

Lentil and Vegetable Soup

Prep time: 15 mins   Cooking: 30 mins   servings:6

Ingredients

- 1 cup green lentils, rinsed
- 1 onion, chopped
- 2 carrots, diced
- 2 celery stalks, sliced
- 4 cups vegetable broth
- 1 teaspoon turmeric
- 1 teaspoon cumin
- Salt and pepper to taste

Instructions

1. In a pot, sauté onions, carrots, and celery until softened.
2. Add lentils, vegetable broth, turmeric, cumin, salt, and pepper. Simmer until lentils are tender.

Nutritional Value (per serving)

- Calories: 220
- Fiber: 12g
- Protein: 14g

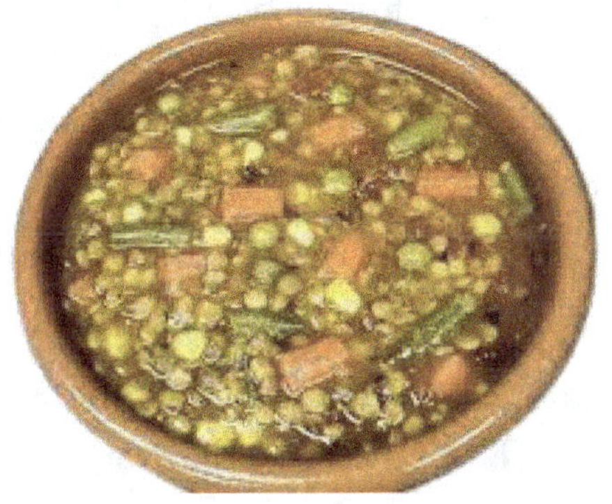

Grilled Chicken and Quinoa Bowl

Prep time: 20 mins   Cooking: 15 mins   servings:4

Ingredients

- grilled apple cider vinegar chicken (16 oz.)
- 1 cup sliced cherry tomatoes 2 cups cooked quinoa
- 1 cup cucumbers, diced
- 1/2 cup drained pickled onions
- 1/2 cup feta cheese, crumbled
- spinach or a mixture of baby greens

- 1/2 cup vinaigrette dressing with lemon

Instructions

1. Once you've prepared all of your ingredients, select four containers and assemble the bowls (I prefer to use rectangular glass storage containers).
2. Top each container with a handful of greens, 4 oz of grilled chicken, 1/2 cup cooked quinoa, 1/4 cup tomatoes and cucumbers, 2 Tablespoons pickled onions, and feta cheese.
3. Divide the dressing into two separate containers for convenient transport. If you want to eat the salads at home, keep the dressing in a bigger container and use as required. I keep mine in a little mason jar.

Nutritional Value (per serving)

- Calories: 380
- Fiber: 8g
- Protein: 30g

Sweet Potato and Chickpea Buddha Bowl

Prep time: 25 mins   Cooking: 30 mins   servings:2

Ingredients

- 2 sweet potatoes, diced
- 1 can (15 oz) chickpeas, drained and rinsed
- 2 cups kale, chopped
- 1/4 cup tahini
- 1 tablespoon olive oil
- 1 teaspoon paprika

Instructions

1. Roast sweet potatoes and chickpeas in olive oil and paprika until golden.
2. Assemble bowls with roasted veggies, kale, and drizzle with tahini.

Nutritional Value (per serving)

- Calories: 420
- Fiber: 12g
- Protein: 15g

Eggplant and Tomato Quinoa Salad

Prep time: 15 mins   Cooking: 20 mins   servings:4

Ingredients

- 1 cup quinoa, cooked
- 1 eggplant, diced
- 1 cup cherry tomatoes, halved
- 1/2 cup red onion, finely chopped
- 1/4 cup fresh basil, chopped
- 3 tablespoons balsamic vinaigrette
- 2 tablespoons olive oil

Instructions

1. Roast the eggplant in olive oil until soft.
2. Combine the quinoa, roasted eggplant, cherry tomatoes, red onion, and basil in a mixing bowl. Drizzle with balsamic vinaigrette and serve.

Nutritional Value (per serving)

- Calories: 320
- Fiber: 8g
- Protein: 9g

Tuna and White Bean Salad

Prep time: 10 mins   Cooking: 0 mins   servings:2

Ingredients

- 2 cans (5 oz each) tuna, drained
- 1 can (15 oz) white beans, drained and rinsed
- 1 cup cherry tomatoes, quartered
- 1/2 cup red bell pepper, diced
- 2 tablespoons red wine vinegar
- 3 tablespoons olive oil
- 1 teaspoon Dijon mustard

Instructions

1. Combine tuna, white beans, cherry tomatoes, and red bell pepper in a mixing bowl.
2. Combine the red wine vinegar, olive oil, and Dijon mustard in a mixing bowl. Toss the salad lightly with the dressing.

Nutritional Value (per serving)

- Calories: 380

- Fiber: 10g
- Protein: 30g

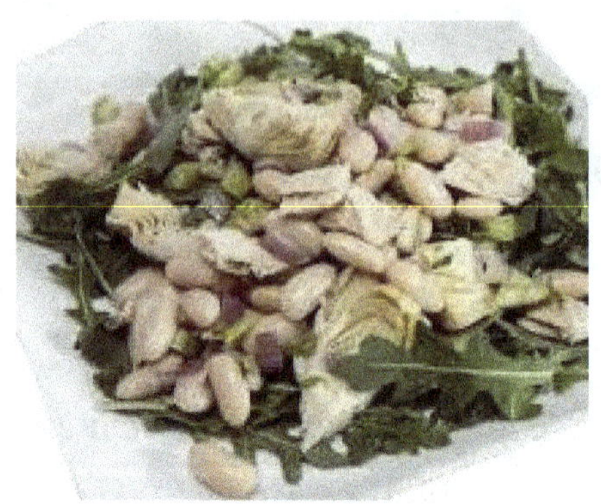

Spinach and Mushroom Quiche

Prep time: 10 mins **Cooking: 0 mins** **servings:6**

Ingredients

- 1 pie crust (whole grain if available)
- 2 cups spinach, chopped
- 1 cup mushrooms, sliced
- 6 eggs
- 1 cup almond milk
- 1/2 cup feta cheese, crumbled
- Salt and pepper to taste

Instructions

1. Preheat the oven to 375 degrees Fahrenheit (190 degrees Celsius).
2. Sauté the spinach and mushrooms until they are wilted. Fill the pie shell halfway with the mixture.
3. Combine the eggs, almond milk, feta, salt, and pepper in a mixing bowl. Pour the sauce over the spinach and mushrooms.
4. Bake until the quiche is brown and firm.

Nutritional Value (per serving)

- Calories: 280
- Fiber: 4g
- Protein: 15g

Brown Rice and Vegetable Stir-Fry

Prep time: 15 mins   Cooking: 20 mins   servings:4

Ingredients

- 2 cups brown rice, cooked
- 1 cup broccoli florets
- 1 cup snap peas

- 1 carrot, julienned
- 1 bell pepper, sliced
- 1 cup tofu, cubed
- 2 tablespoons soy sauce
- 1 tablespoon sesame oil

Instructions

1. In a wok, stir-fry tofu until golden. Add vegetables and cook until crisp-tender.
2. Mix in cooked brown rice, soy sauce, and sesame oil. Stir until well combined.

Nutritional Value (per serving)

- Calories: 340
- Fiber: 8g
- Protein: 12g

Cauliflower and Chickpea Curry

Prep time: 10 mins   Cooking: 0 mins   servings:4

Ingredients

- 1 head cauliflower, cut into florets
- 1 can (15 oz) chickpeas, drained and rinsed
- 1 onion, finely chopped
- 2 tomatoes, diced
- 1 can (14 oz) coconut milk
- 2 tablespoons curry powder
- 1 tablespoon olive oil

Instructions

1. Cook until the onions are transparent in olive oil. After adding the curry powder, cook for another minute.
2. Combine cauliflower, chickpeas, tomatoes, and coconut milk in a mixing bowl. Cook until the cauliflower is soft.

Nutritional Value (per serving)

- Calories: 280
- Fiber: 10g
- Protein: 10g

Dinner

Baked Salmon with Lemon and Herbs

Prep time: 10 mins   Cooking: 20 mins   servings:4

Ingredients

- 4 salmon fillets, skinned (approximately 2 pounds (900g) total)
- 4 cups brussels sprouts, halved
- 2 tablespoons melted unsalted butter
- 2 tbsp fresh rosemary, chopped (or 1 tbsp dried rosemary)
- 2 tablespoons fresh chopped parsley (or 1 tablespoon dry)
- 1 tbsp. minced garlic
- 2 medium lemons, cut in half
- 1/2 teaspoon freshly ground black pepper, to taste, divided sea salt

Instructions

1. Preheat the oven to 400°F (204°C). To line a baking sheet, use parchment paper or a silicone baking mat.

Arrange salmon and brussels sprouts on top, equally spaced.

2. Brush each salmon fillet with melted butter. In a small bowl, combine the rosemary, parsley, garlic, lemon juice (about 4 tablespoons), and 1/4 teaspoon pepper. Spoon equally over each fillet, spreading evenly. Place 1-2 slices of the second lemon on top of each fillet. Squeeze the other half of the lemon over the brussels sprouts. Season the brussels sprouts with the remaining 1/4 teaspoon pepper. Sprinkle sea salt evenly over the entire pan not much is required, but use your discretion.

3. Bake for 15-20 minutes, depending on thickness, or until the thickest section reaches 145°F (63°C) internal heat.

4. Serve hot.

Nutritional Value (per serving)

- Calories: 320
- Fiber: 0g
- Protein: 30g

Vegetarian Chickpea and Spinach Curry

Prep time: 15 mins   Cooking: 25 mins   servings:4

Ingredients

- 1 tablespoon coconut oil
- 1 large or 2 normal onions (optional for a richer sauce) very finely diced
- 3 garlic cloves, minced 400 g cherry tomatoes, roughly halved 2 punnets
- 1 teaspoon garam masala
- 1-12 teaspoon curry powder add extra to increase the heat
- 12 teaspoon turmeric 12 teaspoon powdered cinnamon 14 teaspoon ground cardamom
- 12 teaspoon ground cumin 12 teaspoon sea salt plus more to taste
- 12 teaspoon grated ginger
- 1 tablespoon tomato paste
- 480 g cooked chickpeas, or 2 cans (drained)
- 14 cup vegetable stock or water 200 ml coconut milk half a 400 ml (14 oz) can
- 3 cups fresh baby spinach
- 1 teaspoon chilli flakes or sliced green chilies (optional)

Instructions

1. In a heavy-bottomed saucepan over medium heat, melt the coconut oil and sauté the onion for 3-5 minutes, or until tender.
2. Combine the garlic and tomatoes in a mixing bowl.
3. Combine garam masala, curry powder, turmeric, cinnamon, cardamom, cumin, ginger, tomato paste, and sea salt in a mixing bowl. Cook for another 2 minutes.
4. Stir in the chickpeas to coat them. Bring the coconut milk and vegetable stock to a boil in a saucepan.
5. Reduce the heat to low and simmer for 25-30 minutes, or until the sauce is thick and creamy, with the lid off. Allow the young spinach to wilt gently in the pan.
6. Remove from the fire and serve with a sprinkle of chilli flakes or chiles and cooked rice or quinoa.

Nutritional Value (per serving)

- Calories: 280
- Fiber: 8g
- Protein: 10g

Grilled Turkey and Vegetable Kabobs

Prep time: 20 mins   Cooking: 15 mins   servings:4

Ingredients

- 1 pound turkey breast, cut into cubes
- Bell peppers (assorted colors)
- Cherry tomatoes
- Red onion
- 2 tablespoons olive oil
- 1 teaspoon paprika
- Salt and pepper to taste

Instructions

1. Toss turkey, bell peppers, cherry tomatoes, and red onion with olive oil and paprika in a mixing bowl.
2. Thread the turkey onto skewers and grill until cooked through.

Nutritional Value (per serving)

- Calories: 250
- Fiber: 4g
- Protein: 30g

Quinoa Stuffed Bell Peppers

Prep time: 20 mins   Cooking: 30 mins   servings:4

Ingredients

- 4 bell peppers, halved
- 1 cup quinoa, cooked
- Black beans
- Corn kernels
- 1 cup cherry tomatoes, diced
- 1 teaspoon cumin powder
- 1/2 cup cilantro, chopped

Instructions

1. Preheat the oven to 375°F (190°C).
2. In a bowl, mix quinoa, black beans, corn, cherry tomatoes, cumin powder, and cilantro.
3. Stuff the bell peppers with the quinoa mixture and bake until peppers are tender.

Nutritional Value (per serving)

- Calories: 300
- Fiber: 10g

- Protein: 12g

Mushroom and Spinach Stuffed Chicken Breast

Prep time: 15 mins   Cooking: 30 mins   servings:3

Ingredients

- 2 teaspoons olive oil
- 12 teaspoon Italian Seasoning 1 teaspoon butter 2 garlic cloves chopped 10-12 button mushrooms approx 200 grams, thickly sliced Blend

- 3 skinless (boneless) chicken breasts
- 2 cups coarsely chopped (loosely packed) spinach leaves
- 34 cup grated Mozzarella Salt and pepper

Instructions

1. In a cast iron pan, heat a tablespoon of oil and add the mushrooms and garlic. On high heat, toss the mushrooms with the Italian seasoning mix and salt for 2-3 minutes, or until golden brown and slightly

crispy around the edges. Transfer to a bowl and put aside.

2. Butterfly the chicken (or slice it in half without cutting all the way through) to fill the chicken breasts. The chicken breast should expand out like a butterfly, with one end remaining intact in the middle). Season with salt and pepper on both sides.

3. Now, open the chicken breast so that it resembles a butterfly. Place a spoonful or two of mushrooms on one side, followed by a handful of spinach leaves, and then 14 grated cheese. Fold the other side of the chicken breast on top and seal it with a toothpick to prevent the stuffing from escaping. Repeat with the remaining chicken breasts.

4. In the same pan, heat the remaining oil and butter and add the chicken breasts. Begin on high heat and then decrease to medium after a minute. Cook the breasts for 6-7 minutes on each side, depending on their size. Place on a platter and let aside for 2-3 minutes before serving.

Notes

- How to tell whether the chicken is done: Cooked chicken should have an internal temperature of 165F/73C. A meat thermometer would be the most convenient method to tell. If you don't have one, you can chop and examine the fluids by hand. The chicken is done when the flesh is white in color and the fluids flow clear. The meat or liquids should not be red/pinkish in color.

- For this dish, the chicken must be butterflyed. Use a sharp paring knife to make the cut simpler to perform.
- While the chicken is pan frying, use a spoon to catch the pan juices and pour them back over it. Continue basting it in this manner. This keeps the chicken moist and juicy.

Nutritional Value (per serving)

- Calories: 320
- Fiber: 2g
- Protein: 30g

Lemon Garlic Shrimp and Asparagus

Prep time: 15 mins   Cooking: 10 mins   servings:2

Ingredients

- 1 pound shrimp, peeled and deveined
- Asparagus spears

- 2 tablespoons olive oil
- Garlic cloves, minced
- 1 teaspoon lemon zest
- 1 tablespoon fresh lemon juice
- Salt and pepper to taste

Instructions

1. In a pan, sauté shrimp and asparagus in olive oil until shrimp turn pink and asparagus is tender.
2. Stir in minced garlic, lemon zest, and lemon juice. Season with salt and pepper.

Nutritional Value (per serving)

- Calories: 280
- Fiber: 4g
- Protein: 25g

Sweet Potato and Lentil Curry

Prep time: 20 mins   Cooking: 25 mins   servings:4

Ingredients

- 2 sweet potatoes, diced
- 1 cup green lentils, rinsed
- 1 onion, finely chopped
- 2 tomatoes, diced
- 1 can (14 oz) coconut milk
- 2 tablespoons curry powder
- 1 tablespoon olive oil

Instructions

1. Cook until the onions are transparent in olive oil. Cook for another minute after adding the curry powder.
2. Combine the sweet potatoes, lentils, tomatoes, and coconut milk in a mixing bowl. Cook until the sweet potatoes are soft.

Nutritional Value (per serving)

- Calories: 320
- Fiber: 12g
- Protein: 14g

Cauliflower Rice Stir-Fry with Tofu

Prep time: 15 mins   Cooking: 20 mins   servings:4

Ingredients

- 1 block tofu, cubed
- Cauliflower rice
- 1 cup broccoli florets
- 1 carrot, julienned
- 1 red bell pepper, sliced
- 2 tablespoons soy sauce
- 1 tablespoon sesame oil

Instructions

1. Stir-fry tofu in a wok until browned. Cook until the veggies are crisp-tender.
2. Combine cauliflower rice, soy sauce, and sesame oil in a mixing bowl. Stir until well combined.

Nutritional Value (per serving)

- Calories: 320
- Fiber: 8g
- Protein: 18g

Salmon and Quinoa Stuffed Zucchini

Prep time: 20 mins   Cooking: 25 mins   servings:4

Ingredients

- 4 zucchinis, halved
- 2 salmon fillets, cooked and flaked
- 1 cup quinoa, cooked
- Cherry tomatoes
- 1/4 cup fresh parsley, chopped
- 2 tablespoons olive oil
- Lemon wedges for serving

Instructions

1. Scoop out the center of each zucchini half.
2. In a bowl, mix flaked salmon, quinoa, cherry tomatoes, and parsley. Stuff the zucchinis with the mixture.
3. Drizzle with olive oil and bake until zucchinis are tender.

Nutritional Value (per serving)

- Calories: 350
- Fiber: 6g

- Protein: 25g

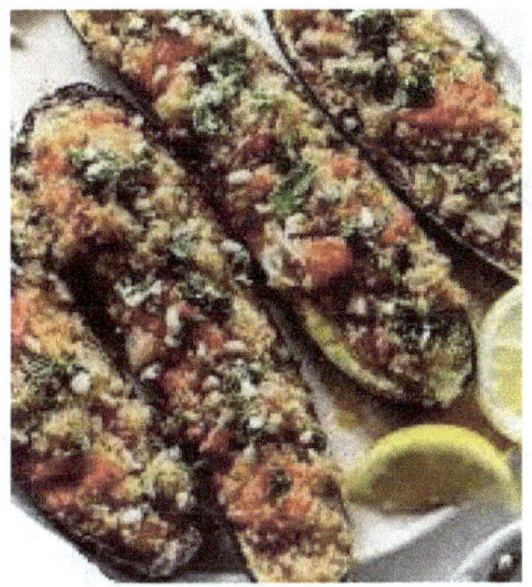

Miso-Glazed Eggplant with Brown Rice

Prep time: 15 mins   Cooking: 25 mins   servings:2

Ingredients

- 2 eggplants, sliced
- Brown rice, cooked
- 2 tablespoons miso paste
- 1 tablespoon maple syrup
- 1 tablespoon rice vinegar
- 1 teaspoon sesame oil
- Sesame seeds for garnish

Instructions

1. Preheat the oven to 400 degrees Fahrenheit (200 degrees Celsius).
2. In a mixing bowl, combine miso paste, maple syrup, rice vinegar, and sesame oil.
3. Brush the eggplant slices with the miso glaze and bake until soft.
4. Sprinkle with sesame seeds and serve over brown rice.

Nutritional Value (per serving)

- Calories: 300
- Fiber: 8g
- Protein: 6g

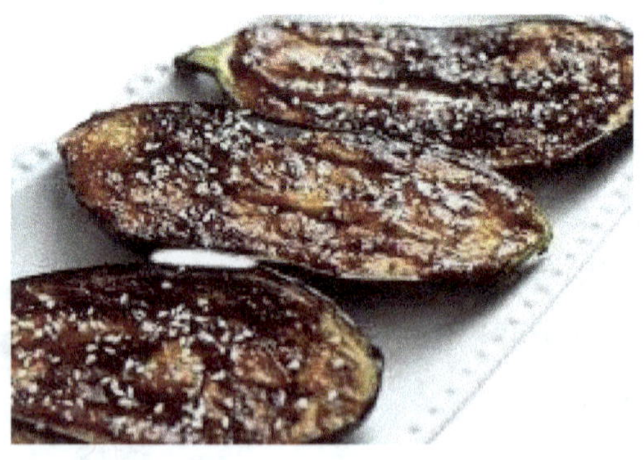

Snacks

Turmeric Roasted Chickpeas

Prep time: 5 mins   Cooking: 30 mins   servings:4

Ingredients

- 2 cans (15 oz each) drained and washed chickpeas
- 2 tbsp of olive oil
- 1 teaspoon powdered turmeric
- a half teaspoon cumin
- 1 tablespoon smoked paprika
- Season with salt to taste

Instructions

1. Preheat the oven to 400°F (200 degrees Celsius).
2. Toss chickpeas with olive oil, turmeric, cumin, smoked paprika, and salt in a mixing bowl.
3. Roast the chickpeas on a baking sheet until brown and crispy.

Nutritional Value (per serving)

- Calories: 180
- Fiber: 8g

- Protein: 7g

Avocado and Tomato Salsa with Whole Grain Crackers

Prep time: 10 mins   **Cooking: 0 mins**   **servings:2**

Ingredients

- 2 diced avocados
- 1 cup chopped cherry tomatoes
- 1/4 cup coarsely chopped red onion
- 1/4 cup chopped fresh cilantro
- Serve with whole grain crackers.
- 1 tablespoon extra virgin olive oil
- One lime juice
- Season with salt and pepper to taste.

Instructions

1. Combine avocados, tomatoes, red onion, and cilantro in a mixing dish.
2. Drizzle with olive oil and lime juice to finish. Season with salt and pepper to taste.
3. With whole grain crackers, serve.

Nutritional Value (per serving)

- Calories: 220
- Fiber: 8g
- Protein: 4g

Greek Yogurt and Berry Parfait

Prep time: 7 mins   Cooking: 0 mins   servings:2

Ingredients

- 1 cup plain Greek yogurt
- 1/2 cup blueberries, strawberries, and raspberries
- 2 teaspoons honey 1/4 cup chopped almonds
- a half teaspoon of vanilla extract

Instructions

1. Layer Greek yogurt, mixed berries, and sliced almonds in glasses.
2. Drizzle honey over the top and sprinkle with vanilla essence.

Nutritional Value (per serving)

- Calories: 280
- Fiber: 6g
- Protein: 14g

Kale Chips

Prep time: 10 mins   Cooking: 15 mins   servings:4

Ingredients

- 1 bunch kale, stems removed and torn into pieces
- 2 tablespoons olive oil
- 1 teaspoon turmeric powder
- 1/2 teaspoon garlic powder
- Salt to taste

Instructions

- Preheat the oven to 350°F (175°C).
- In a bowl, massage kale with olive oil, turmeric, garlic powder, and salt.
- Spread kale on a baking sheet and bake until crisp.

Nutritional Value (per serving)

- Calories: 60
- Fiber: 2g
- Protein: 2g

Chia Pudding with Mango

Prep time: 5 mins   Cooking: 0 mins   servings:2

Ingredients

- 1 tablespoon chia seeds
- 1-quart almond milk
- 1 teaspoon powdered turmeric
- 1 diced ripe mango
- 2 tbsp of coconut flakes

Instructions

1. Combine the chia seeds, almond milk, and turmeric in a mixing dish. Refrigerate until it approaches the consistency of pudding.
2. In glasses, layer chia pudding with chopped mango.
3. Sprinkle with coconut flakes.

Nutritional Value (per serving)

- Calories: 220
- Fiber: 12g
- Protein: 5g

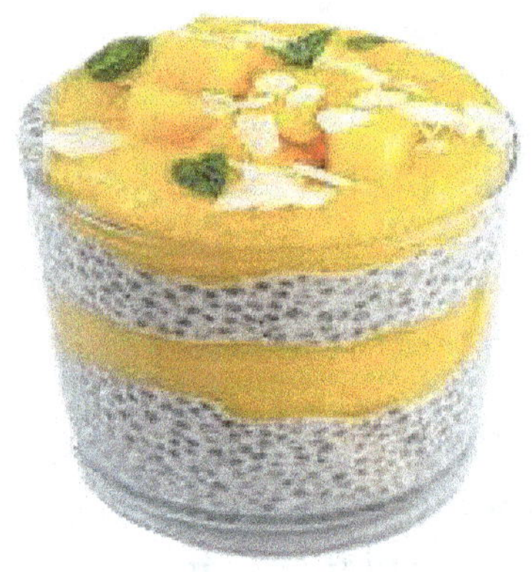

Chapter 5: Mastering Intermittent

Exploring different intermittent fasting schedules: 16:8, 5:2, and beyond.

Intermittent fasting (IF) has grown in popularity as a technique for weight loss, metabolic health, and general well-being. Within the context of the Galveston Diet, IF provides a flexible way to optimizing your eating window and properly fueling your body. This chapter goes into several IF schedules, allowing you to pick one that fits your lifestyle and tastes.

The 16:8 Method:

The Lean Gains technique, often known as the 16:8 approach, entails a 16-hour fast followed by an 8-hour eating window during a 24-hour period. This is how it works:

Fasting Window (16 Hours): This encompasses the majority of your sleep as well as some awake hours. During this period, stick to water, unsweetened tea, and black coffee.

Eating Window (8 Hours): Eat all of your meals and snacks inside this time frame. Eat anti-inflammatory, nutrient-dense meals first, and eat intuitively in response to hunger cues.

The 16:8 technique is an easy way to get started with IF, especially for novices. Its adaptability allows for social interactions as well as different eating timings.

The 5:2 Method

The 5:2 technique is eating regularly for five days and limiting calories to 500-600 on two non-consecutive days per week. You may organize your fasting days as you want:

Complete Fast: During the day of fasting, only drink water, black coffee, and unsweetened tea.

Modified Fast: On fasting days, consume one modest meal and one or two tiny snacks.

This strategy provides flexibility for people with hectic schedules who may find daily fasting difficult. Remember to prioritize healthy foods on non-fasting days to compensate for lower calorie intake on fasting days.

Beyond the Common Protocols

Two examples are the 16:8 and 5:2 techniques. Several additional IF schedules can be tailored to your requirements:

Eat-Stop-Eat: Once or twice a week, fast for 24 hours.

Fasting every other day is known as alternate-day fasting.

Feeding on a Timer: Choose a shorter eating window, such as 12:12 or 10:14.

Tips for navigating social events, travel, and unexpected situations.

Embracing the Galveston Diet does not imply foregoing these events; rather, it means arming yourself with the tools to traverse them gracefully while remaining committed to your health objectives. So, bring your resilience, a pinch of flexibility, and let's talk about how to conquer social events, travel like a gastronomic adventurer, and negotiate unexpected times with confidence.

Social Gatherings

Dieters may find dinner parties, weddings, and informal get-togethers to be minefields. But don't worry, future socialite! Your hidden weapons are as follows:

Planning Ability: If feasible, research meals ahead of time. Look for anti-inflammatory foods such as grilled fish, roasted vegetables, and salads that may be customized.

Bring a buddy: Bring a sympathetic buddy who knows your food preferences. They may be your wingman, guiding you to healthier selections and sharing in your delight.

Portion Control: Remember that attentive eating is essential. Enjoy modest quantities of tasty foods, prevent mindless munching, and put quality over quantity first.

Hydration Hero: Throughout the event, sip on water or sparkling water. It keeps you full, assists you in making conscious decisions, and avoids alcohol-induced cravings.

Dessert Diplomacy: Avoid sugary bombshells in favor of fruit-based sweets, a modest piece of dark chocolate, or a cup of herbal tea. Remember that you may always gently refuse an enticing offer.

Travel Tales

Exploring new landscapes frequently entails discovering new gastronomic vistas. Don't allow your Galveston Diet journey be derailed by travel; instead, make it into a delightful experience!

Stock Your Pantry: Pack travel-friendly foods like almonds, seeds, dried fruit, and protein bars in your luggage. They'll be useful on lengthy travels or when healthful alternatives are scarce.

Market Marvels: Visit local markets and look for fresh, seasonal goods. Grilled meats, vibrant salads, and whole-grain foods are all good choices. Embrace your destination's tastes!

Restaurant Research: Look for eateries that include anti-inflammatory alternatives on their menus. Don't be afraid to request changes, such as omitting sauces or opting for grilled rather than fried items.

Preparing Skills: If you live in an apartment, think about purchasing groceries and preparing some meals yourself. You have total control over the components and portion quantities.

Embrace Cultural Cuisine: Many cuisines from throughout the world are inherently anti-inflammatory, with a high concentration of spices, veggies, and healthy fats. Discover amazing hidden gems and local specialties!

Unexpected Encounters

Life throws curveballs, and healthy options might feel restricted at times. But keep in mind that your strength is resilience!

The Late-Night Craving: Keep healthful snacks on hand, such as berries, yogurt, or hard-boiled eggs, for those unexpected moments. They'll satisfy your appetites without jeopardizing your ambitions.

The Restaurant Rendezvous: Give veggies and protein the highest priority when there aren't many alternatives. Order a grilled chicken salad instead of fish, and ask for steamed veggies on the side.

The Social Mistake: Don't punish yourself for occasional indiscretions. Enjoy them attentively, return to your next meal, and remember that growth, not perfection, is the goal.

The Holiday Extravaganza: The holidays are about having fun, not feeling guilty. Consume holiday parties in moderation, practice mindful eating, and select healthy options at other meals.

Pay Attention to Your Body: Pay attention to your body's cues during all of these scenarios. Stop eating when you're satisfied, and remember that tiny, regular actions contribute to long-term development.

Social gatherings, travel, and unforeseen occurrences are not impediments; they are chances to exhibit your dedication to your health. Applying these principles and adopting a flexible mentality will make negotiating these circumstances simpler with each experience. Remember that the Galveston Diet is a compass that will lead you to a healthier, happier, and more vibrant existence. So, pack your fortitude, adventurous spirit, and newfound knowledge, and embark on the thrilling voyage ahead!

Overcoming hunger cravings and staying motivated during fasting periods.

First, let's debunk the myth of hunger. Contrary to common opinion, fasting hunger is often caused by our body adapting to a new eating pattern rather than by a lack of immediate nourishment. It's a typical physiological response that usually peaks in the first few days and eventually fades as your body adapts.

Let us now empower you with techniques for fending off the hungry tiger:

Hydration Hero: Your secret weapon is water. Thirst may frequently be confused with hunger, so have a glass nearby and drink throughout the day. A delightful zing may be added to sparkling water with a squeeze of lemon or cucumber.

Distraction Dynamo: Use your brain! Take a stroll, read a book, listen to music, or phone a friend. Distraction breaks the hunger cycle and shifts your attention away from your stomach.

Herbal Haven: Drink herbal teas such as ginger, peppermint, or chamomile. These include natural hunger suppressants and give a nice, warm sensation.

Mindful Movement: Gentle exercise, such as yoga or strolling, can increase the release of endorphins, which improve mood and reduce perceived hunger.

Sleep Sanctuary: Make sleep a priority! When you don't get enough sleep, your body creates more ghrelin, the hunger hormone. Aim for 7-8 hours of excellent sleep every night to keep your hunger at bay.

Chapter 7: Conquering Challenges and Roadblocks

Addressing weight plateaus, hormonal fluctuations, and social setbacks.

Your journey, like any other, will not be without incident. Weight plateaus, hormone changes, and social disappointments will all test your resolve. These might be disappointing, leaving you feeling befuddled and unsure of your progress. But don't worry, daring explorer! This will provide you with the tools and resilience you need to traverse these turbulent waters and emerge triumphant, your spirit unafraid and your objective in sight.

Weight Plateau Purgatory

The dreaded plateau - a period in which your weight loss stops, leaving you disappointed and questioning your efforts. But keep in mind that losing weight is not a straight line. Your body, like any other complex ecosystem, is adjusting to new habits and fuel sources. Here's how to get out of plateau purgatory:

Change Your Focus: Stop obsessing over the scale. Celebrate non-scale wins like as more energy, better sleep, and better clothing fit.

Incorporate diversity into your workouts. Try high-intensity interval exercise, weight training, or even dancing in your living room! Keep your body guessing and your metabolism going.

Analyze your meal choices and fuel yourself wisely. Are you unintentionally introducing hidden sweets or bad fats? Prioritize nutrient-dense, anti-inflammatory meals and watch your servings.

Hydration Hero: Your secret weapon is water. Dehydration can cause weight reduction to halt. Aim for eight glasses of water every day and your body will reward you.

Seek Help: Consult your doctor or a qualified nutritionist. They can analyze your progress and provide tailored advice to help you break through the plateau.

Hormonal Disorders

With its shifting hormones, menopause may send your metabolism into overdrive. But remember, even in the midst of this emotional tempest, you have the ability to remain anchored. Here's how to deal with the hormonal upheaval:

Prioritize sleep in your sleep sanctuary. When you don't get enough sleep, your body creates more cortisol, a stress hormone that stifles weight loss. Each night, aim for 7-8 hours of decent sleep.

Stress Management: Manage stress by practicing yoga, meditation, or spending time in nature. Chronic stress can aggravate hormone abnormalities and stymie growth.

Mindful Movement: Regular exercise is a must. Even modest action, such as walking or yoga, can help balance hormones and improve your mood.

Focus on anti-inflammatory foods including fruits, vegetables, and healthy fats. These aid in hormone balance and general well-being.

Seek Help: Do not go it alone. Connect with other women going through menopause. Share your stories, advice, and words of support. Remember that you are not alone in this.

Social Setbacks

Birthdays, holidays, and social gatherings may all be traps for good intentions. However, with the right methods, you can negotiate these minefields without jeopardizing your development. Here's how to recover from social setbacks:

Prepare ahead of time: Before attending an event, look into food alternatives or carry healthy snacks. Having a strategy eliminates impulsive, harmful decisions.

Enjoy social occasions without starving yourself by practicing mindful moderation. Savour little amounts of goodies and emphasize healthful options throughout the day.

Positive Reframing: Look at failures as chances to learn. Determine what set you off and devise tactics to prevent such circumstances in the future.

Self-Compassion: Don't be too hard on yourself! Dwelling on mistakes just slows down growth. Forgive yourself, get back on track, and rejoice in your overall accomplishments.

Celebrate Non-Scale Victories: Think positively! Did you resist the urge to overeat? Did you prefer water over sugary drinks? Celebrate your minor successes!

Maintaining commitment and motivation in the long run

Motivation, like a flickering flame, requires regular attention to stay lit. Here are some ideas for reigniting your enthusiasm and staying committed:

Remember Your "Why": Reconnect with the fundamental motivations that led you on this path. Is it bettering your health, increasing your energy, or making you feel more confident in your body? Keep your "why" at the forefront of your mind, especially when motivation wanes.

Non-Scale Victories Should Be Celebrated: Concentrate on the improvement rather than the number on the scale. Celebrate renewed energy, better sleep, better clothing fit, or a newfound enthusiasm for fresh fruit.

Discover Your Tribe: Surround yourself with individuals who are encouraging and supportive of your health objectives. Join online communities, find a gym companion, or connect with other people who share your interests. Their words of support and shared experiences will keep you motivated.

Small Steps, Massive Strides: Remember that little, consistent steps lead to long-term progress. Don't stress yourself out by making big adjustments. Set attainable daily or weekly objectives and celebrate every success, no matter how little.

Accept Imperfections: Don't allow little blunders hinder your development. Consider them learning experiences and get back on track with your next meal. Self-compassion and forgiveness are essential for long-term motivation.

Overcoming the Motivational Hill

On a lengthy journey, even the most devoted trekker may experience exhaustion. Here are some strategies for overcoming motivational lows:

Keep things interesting: Variety is the spice of life! Experiment with fresh foods, varied fitness regimens, and healthy methods to satisfy cravings. Keeping your excitement alive by avoiding monotony.

Look for Inspiration: Read books or articles on people's journeys to health and wellness. Play podcasts or inspiring lectures. Reading encouraging, inspiring stories might help you rekindle your own light.

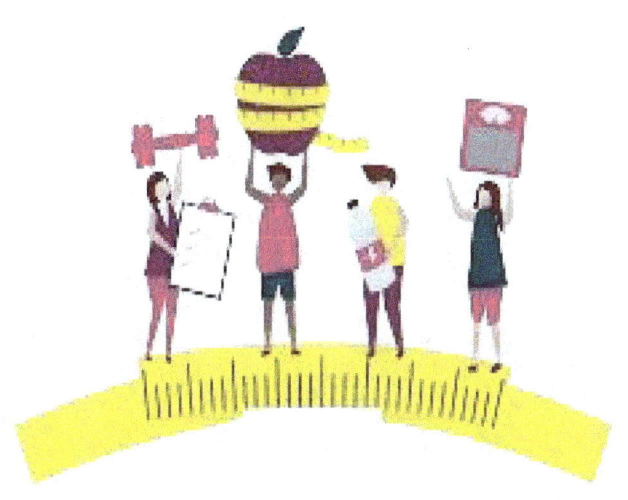

Imagine Your Success: Consider attaining your objectives while feeling bright and healthy. Keep that image in mind throughout difficult times. Visualization may be a very effective strategy for keeping motivated.

Reward Yourself: Celebrate your accomplishments! Get a massage, a weekend vacation, or a new fitness wardrobe. Self-rewarding fosters great behavior and keeps you interested in the path.

Gratitude Practice: Set aside time each day to acknowledge your progress, no matter how tiny. Gratitude redirects your attention to the positive and boosts your enthusiasm to keep going.

Chapter 7: Sustainable Strategies for Maintaining Momentum

Practical Tips for Everyday Life.

The Galveston Diet is a colorful trek toward a lifetime of well-being, not a race to the finish line. It's about incorporating anti-inflammatory ideas into your daily life, adjusting them to your changing requirements, and cultivating a caring connection with oneself along the way. This provides you with the practical skills and conscious mentality you need to keep your momentum going, convert the Galveston Diet into your new normal, and lay the groundwork for healthy aging that radiates energy through every decade.

Incorporate the Galveston Diet concepts into your everyday routine, making them as automatic as brushing your teeth:

Embrace the Power of Planning: Plan your meals and snacks in advance to ensure you have access to healthy alternatives throughout the day. Anti-inflammatory essentials like fruits, veggies, nutritious grains, and lean meats should be in your cupboard.

Become a Kitchen Alchemist: Explore diverse cuisines and flavors by experimenting with new dishes within the Galveston framework. Cooking at home allows you to manage the ingredients and portion amounts, which helps you stay on track.

Make Friends with Batch Cooking: Make huge amounts of healthful meals on weekends or evenings to save time throughout the week. Soups, stews, and roasted veggies are good choices for quick, healthy dinners.

Mindful Grocery Shopping: Make educated decisions in the grocery aisle. Read labels carefully, favor healthy foods over processed goods, and buy locally and seasonally wherever feasible.

Become a Label Detective: Learn how to easily interpret food labels. Identify hidden sugars and harmful fats, and prioritize fiber, vitamin, and mineral-rich meals.

Dine Confidently: Navigate restaurant menus with ease. Look for grilled, baked, or steamed alternatives, prioritize protein and veggies, and don't be afraid to request dietary changes.

Hydration Superstar: Always keep a reusable water bottle with you. Aim for eight glasses of water each day, and for a taste boost, try herbal teas or infused water.

Joyfully Move Your Body: Find an exercise program that you love, whether it's going for brisk walks, dancing in your living room, or signing up for a fitness class. Make activity a habit rather than a chore.

Sleep should be prioritized: Aim for 7-8 hours of excellent sleep every night. Set a consistent sleep schedule, develop a calming evening ritual, and minimize screen time before bed.

Make Stress Your Friend: Stress can be reduced by practicing mindfulness meditation, yoga, spending time in nature, or connecting with loved ones. Chronic stress can stymie growth and have a detrimental influence on your well-being.

Adapting the Journey to the Stages of Life

The Galveston Diet does not apply to everyone. It may be tailored to your specific needs and life stages:

Younger Adults: Concentrate on developing lifelong healthy habits, learning to make nutritious meals, and laying a solid foundation of physical exercise.

Growing Families: Tailor recipes and meal planning to children's tastes, get them involved in the kitchen, and make family meals a time for connection and healthy choices.

Pregnant and Breastfeeding Women: Prioritize nutrient-rich meals to assist both mother and baby, get particular dietary advice from a doctor or trained dietitian, and pay attention to your body's changing requirements.

Menopause and Beyond: Adapt your diet to hormonal shifts, emphasize foods high in calcium and vitamin D that are good for your bones, and get moving to keep your weight under control and your mental health intact.

Laying the Groundwork for Healthy Aging

As you become older, the Galveston Diet principles become increasingly more important. They provide a road map for good aging by encouraging energy and independence:

Prioritize Plant Power: To battle inflammation and boost cognitive function, eat colorful fruits and vegetables high in antioxidants and fiber.

Embrace Healthy Fats: Include heart-healthy fats in your diet, such as olive oil, avocado, and almonds, to safeguard your heart and brain health.

Strengthen Your Bones: Get enough calcium and vitamin D to keep your bones strong and avoid osteoporosis. After checking with your doctor, consider daily supplementation.

Keep Hydrated: Dehydration can aggravate age-related health problems. Drink enough of water throughout the day to keep your body operating at peak efficiency.

Move Your Body: Regular physical exercise, even if it's only a simple walk, is vital for maintaining muscle mass, bone density, and general health.

Nurture Your Mind: Engage in brain-stimulating activities such as reading, playing games, or acquiring new skills. This keeps your mind sharp and prevents cognitive deterioration.

Accept Social Connection: Loneliness may be harmful to one's health. Develop strong social links, spend time with loved ones, and engage in things that offer you delight.

CONCLUSION

The journey we've taken together, through the ups and downs of perimenopause and the calmer seas of menopause, isn't about achieving a destination. It's about transformation, about discarding old stories and blossoming into the colorful woman you were always intended to be.

This isn't a tale of dwindling flowers and muted sunsets. It's a transformational symphony in which hot flashes become sparks of inner fire, weight reduction becomes a dance of release, and sleep becomes a source of fresh vitality.

We've explored into the anti-inflammatory dietary secrets, the freeing dance of Intermittent Fasting, and the wisdom of listening to your body's individual demands. We've built a raft of self-compassion, navigated emotional currents, and discovered the joy of movement and mindful living.

But now, my fellow traveler, it's time to abandon the raft. Step onto the beach, feel the warm sand beneath your feet, and inhale the salty air of opportunity. This is your island, illuminated by the bright light of your own brilliance.

Here, you may laugh uncontrollably, dance in the rain without an umbrella, and face the world with renewed vigor. The floods of knowledge and self-care have washed away the whispers of doubt. Fears of aging have vanished in the bright seas of acceptance.

You are the phoenix that has risen from the ashes, your feathers flaming with vivid health and delight. You are the reawakened goddess, recovering your power and spreading it to the world. You are the woman who blooms beyond the bloom, defying expectations and redefining the menopausal narrative.

So, darling sister, go out. With outstretched arms, embrace the planet, your laughter booming across the seas. Allow your story to be a source of hope and inspiration for those who are on their own journeys. This is your moment, your season to shine, to blossom with a ferocity that defies the passage of time and the numbers on a scale.

This is your beautiful menopause. Accept it. Own it. Allow your blossom to become a wildfire, illuminating the path for future generations of women.

CALORIE INTAKE TRACKER

Day	Breakfast	Lunch	Dinner	Snack
SUN				
MON				
TUE				
WED				
THU				
FRI				
SAT				

CALORIE INTAKE TRACKER

Day	Breakfast	Lunch	Dinner	Snack
SUN				
MON				
TUE				
WED				
THU				
FRI				
SAT				

CALORIE INTAKE TRACKER

Day	Breakfast	Lunch	Dinner	Snack
SUN				
MON				
TUE				
WED				
THU				
FRI				
SAT				

CALORIE INTAKE TRACKER

Day	Breakfast	Lunch	Dinner	Snack
SUN				
MON				
TUE				
WED				
THU				
FRI				
SAT